care

for

caregivers

Dr. Roy W. Harris

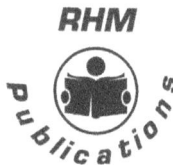

While reading an early draft of *Caring for the Caregiver*, I discovered pages so beautifully written they took my breath away. The chapters buzz with reality and helpful suggestions, written with the insight of a man who has been there. This is a resource volume every pastor will want in his library. If you *know* a caregiver, hand him a copy of this book; it's a how-to course on coming to terms with life's most difficult crises. If you *become* a caregiver, study this book; it's a blueprint on keeping your balance when life turns upside down. If you ever *need* a caregiver, read this book carefully; it will help you appreciate those who rearrange their lives to care for you.

—**Dr. Jack Williams**, director of communications, Free Will Baptist Bible College; editor, *Contact Magazine*

I remember meeting Roy for the first time. I was impressed with his quiet manner yet the stride of a man who had been seasoned by life. I soon came to understand why. As he told his story about the struggle he and his wife had gone through, I thought to myself, there are so many others who are giving care who need to hear this story. I was both pleased and excited when I received an early draft of *Caring for the Caregiver*. Once I began reading the book, I couldn't put it down. This book is a must for every, care giver, pastor, choir director, health care worker, and any- one who wants to better understand how to help and encourage caregivers. Thanks Roy...Many people will be helped and encouraged by this book.

- **Dr. Stan Toler** served as a general superintendent in the Church of the Nazarene and as a pastor in Ohio, Florida, Tennessee, and Oklahoma. Dr. Toler has written more than 100 books selling over 3 million copies worldwide.

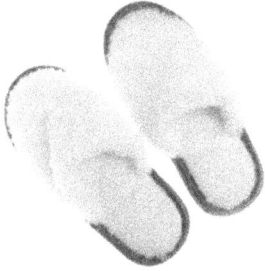

Table of Contents

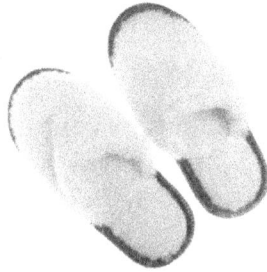

introduction

One of the most traumatic times in life is the loss of a loved one—husband, wife, child, parent, sister, brother, grandparent, or grandchild. Sometimes death comes suddenly, without warning. Other times it approaches like a slow-moving evening shadow. No matter how it arrives, death is always accompanied by a far-reaching, often devastating impact.

Books have been written to comfort and aid those facing death. These resources ease the suffering experienced by those facing terminal illness, and rightly so. These individuals deserve all the help and comfort we can give them. Books have also been written to comfort those who have lost loved ones and help with the grieving process. These books are also needed.

However, one group of individuals is overlooked: the caregivers. They are not overlooked intentionally. By the nature of their role, they are content to stay in the shadow of their loved ones, focused on the needs of the seriously ill or dying. They move quietly through the death process, providing and comforting as they go. Content to lay aside their own feelings, hurts, wants, and needs, they make the waning days as pleasant as possible. These individuals often feel isolated and alone, but they remain strong for the sake of those around them.

In spite of their courage, caregivers desperately need encouragement, comfort, appreciation, love, and a helping hand during this difficult time. This brief book will address those things. Penned by a caregiver who stood faithfully by his wife's side for three years, watching cancer slowly ravage her body and ultimately take her life; the author has firsthand knowledge of a caregiver's experience. He shares practical suggestions to help other caregivers survive emotion- ally. This book will:

• Give practical ways to recognize and cope with different stages of illness

- Provide helpful information about medical terms, procedures, and treatments

- Offer suggestions on how to remain emotionally, spiritually, and physically healthy

- Cite ways to identify and accept outside help from family and friends

- Help family and friends understand what caregivers experience and suggest ways to help and encourage them.

- Suggest personal steps to work through the grieving process

- Give help for the present and hope for the future

More than anything else, the book reminds caregivers that no matter how dark the way may seem, God is still there. No matter how dim the future may look, he is there. No matter what one must endure, he is there. He is there no matter how emotionally wounded one might feel. He gives hope. He offers help. Caregivers can be happy again.

Look to his Word.

I will lift up my eyes to the hills. Where shall my help come from? My help comes from the Lord, who made Heaven and earth. He will not allow your foot to be moved; he who keeps you will not slumber. Behold, he who keeps Israel shall neither slumber nor sleep. The Lord is your keeper; the Lord is your shade on your right hand. The sun shall not strike you by day, nor the moon by night. The Lord shall keep you from all evil; he shall keep your soul. The Lord shall keep your going out and your coming in from this time forth, and even forevermore. Psalm 121 (nkjv)

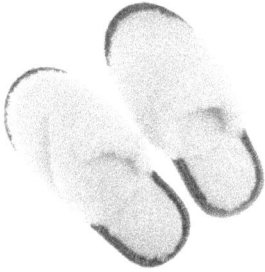

when your world turns upside down

It's amazing how good life is! We often take it for granted, distracted by day-to-day problems that seem large until events change our perspective about what truly is important. The mortgage, kids, car, plumbing, and more weigh heavy on the scale of importance until the scale suddenly tips dramatically in the opposite direction. We forget the importance of health, relationships, and many other good things that God has brought into our lives. We simply take life for granted as routine weaves one day into the next.

I was one of the most blessed men on earth. I had it all multiple college degrees, great ministry, nice home, new car, a beautiful and godly wife, two ne children, and two wonderful grandchildren. While I felt blessed, I did not realize how blessed I was. In a matter of days, however, my stable, ideal world turned upside down.

Diana, my wife, had experienced pain in her left breast. Something was not right. I urged her to make an appointment with her doctor immediately. During the visit, the doctor told us her symptoms could be a sign of something serious. She quickly made Diana an appointment with Dr. Dunbar, a well-known surgeon and specialist in women's health. Dr. Dunbar arranged for a biopsy, and we waited anxiously three days for the results.

The call came on a Monday evening a few minutes after eight. We had just returned home from a pleasant meal with Diana's office staff. I answered the phone. When Dr. Dunbar's voice asked quietly, "Is Diana there," I handed the cordless phone to her and listened closely to her conversation with the doctor. I sensed the news was not good. She hung up the phone and uttered three little words that would change our lives forever: "I have cancer," and she began to cry. I took her in my arms and wept with her. I told her how much I loved her and that we would face this together.

Diana retired early that evening. I normally went to bed an hour or so after her. This night was different. It was not because of needing less sleep that I was awake. I remember so well the emotions of that night.

I require very little sleep. It was a time to be still and reflect over what had just taken place. There are no words to describe my feelings. There were more questions than answers. I could not think of a single person to call who might help with some of those answers. It was late at night and not a good time to call anyone anyway. The only one I could talk to was God himself. This news was devastating. I'm so glad that God never "sleeps or slumbers." The only place I knew to turn was to him.

As I look back on that evening, in some ways it seems long ago. In other ways, it seems like yesterday. Much has happened since that night, but sometimes it is good to look back and remember. I felt so helpless. For more than thirty years, I protected my wife. On that night, I faced something I knew little about, something I couldn't x. Diana looked to me for strength, reassurance, and guidance. I knew I had to remain strong for her and the entire family.

It was hard for me to admit, but I knew this thing was much bigger than I was. In our independent- minded culture, it's hard to admit that we cannot solve every problem. I learned through this experience that it is okay to admit to oneself that there are some things you cannot handle alone. It is hard to admit that we need help, but the sooner we recognize it, the sooner we can accept the help that is available and offered.

The emotions that followed the news were almost unbearable. We had so many questions without answers. *What kind of treatment is available? Can she be cured? Has the cancer spread? Is this disease terminal? How long does she have to live?*

I did not have answers to those questions, but one thing I did know for sure. For thirty years God had blessed our lives together. He had provided every need and taken better care of us than we could have taken ourselves. He had proven his trustworthiness time and time again. What else could we do? I remember thinking of Job in the Bible. Job reached a point when seemingly he lost almost everything that meant anything to him. Even in his despair, Job recognized God's trustworthiness. He said in Job 13:15, "Though he slay me, yet will I trust him" (kjv).

I did not know the answers. I did not even know

all the questions we might have yet. But I came to the realization that I could trust God with my life and the lives of those I cared about.

I didn't realize how blessed I had been until my world changed with one phone call. Three little words changed everything. Faith is a wonderful thing, and it is easy to have faith when your world is filled with good things.

How does faith work when life seems to be getting out of control? I never asked God why this had happened. I must confess, I did tell him that I did not understand. I thought back over my life up to this point. There were other incidents, none as serious as this one, when God seemed to be directing in ways that I did not understand. But in the end, his direction was by far the best direction for my life. He never made a mistake. The strength of his past record with me helped me to go to him with the security of knowing that he knew what he was doing and would not make a mistake with me and my family. For me, the true test of faith began with the ring of that telephone.

Everyone will face a dark day that will reveal the true depth of his or her faith. Some situations are God sized, far too large for us to x. What should we do when our world turns upside down? I remember my words to Diana: "We are placing you in God's hands. I trust him, and I know he will help us." This was the first time I said these words to her, but it would not be the last. These words would be repeated in my mind and orally to her and others many times over the next three years.

We experienced a wonderful peace that could have come only from God. That peace came through a deep held belief that every person is special in God's eyes, a belief that every person is created as a unique human being, designed by God himself with a special purpose and plan for his or her life. Through our experience of living his plan in our lives up to that point and enjoying all his blessings in the past, we believed that his plan was the best plan. We did not know how difficult it might become, but we believed that he was in control.

I remember quoting a verse to myself from the Bible that said "I will never leave you nor forsake you," and another that said "I will be with you even unto the end of the world." What a comfort to know that he was with me and I was not alone. He promised to help me. I knew and believed he would.

Caregiver Principles

- When devastating news comes, place it in God's hands.

- Admit to yourself that you simply cannot handle some things alone.

- Go to him with the security of knowing he does not make mistakes.

- Recognize that you can trust him with life itself and the lives of those you love.

- Believe in your heart that God has a plan for your life.

- It is the best plan, even when it is painful, difficult, and hard to understand.

- Remember: He is in control. He will help you.

fear of the unknown

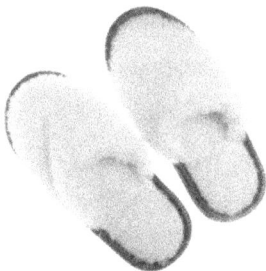

The week seemed endless.
We waited impatiently for Diana's appointment with
the surgeon to find out what "you have cancer" really
meant. I remember watching the Jerry Springer show
in the waiting area. For obvious reasons, I had never
seen a single episode until that day. I would see
several in the coming years because our afternoon
appointments were scheduled so that Diana would
not have to miss work. During those visits, I got a
full taste of so-called reality TV.

When it seemed we could wait no longer, the
door to the inner office swung open and the nurse
called Diana's name. We walked down a winding
hallway to the second examination room on the right.

There was an uneasiness that accompanied each
step we took. Not knowing is one of the hardest
emotions to deal with. I knew what Diana had heard
on the phone. Ever since we received the news, I had
been thinking deep within, wondering just how
serious this might be. I thought of a number of things

the doctor might say. As we passed through the door into the examination room, I knew that the coming minutes could be some of the most important ones that we would ever experience.

Diana insisted that I stay with her for the entire examination. I realized afresh how important it was for my wife to feel secure and not alone. I was glad that I complied with her request. Sometimes the terminally ill loved one is so overwhelmed and confused by the seriousness of what is going on around them that they can fail to fully grasp the diagnosis, possible treatment options, possible side effects of treatment, etc. It was good for me to be in the room and hear all that the doctor had to say.

Dr. Dunbar checked the biopsy incisions then sat down on a swivel stool beside the examining table. As she began sharing the results of the biopsy, we could hardly believe our ears. Not one, but several samples of tissue from the biopsy contained cancerous cells. The cancer was probably present throughout most of the left breast.

With compassionate words and actions, Dr. Dunbar moved from results of the biopsy to bigger issues. Although she was considerate, the news was devastating. She described the tumor as massive.

Surgery was not an option. The tumor was so large it might already be imbedded in the inner chest wall. If this were true, she offered little hope of remission and recovery.

"Just how bad is it?" Diana asked.

Dr. Dunbar explained that the cancer was a fast-growing type with four categories, or stages, with stage four being the most serious. Quietly she said, "Your tumor is already at stage four."

I could not look at Diana. I stared at the floor. My heart was in my throat, and tears filled my eyes. I told myself, *You must keep control. Diana needs you right now.* It was difficult not to break down and weep. As a pastor, I had been in rooms with folks when they received devastating news. This was different.

The doctor explained that patients with Diana's type of cancer usually could expect to live a maximum of eighteen months. The quiet words slowly burned into my mind. We could expect Diana to live no longer than a year and a half. I suddenly felt as though I was trapped in a nightmare and couldn't wake up. I was numb. It was as though someone had knocked all the breath from my lungs. I heard the words, but I could not respond to the voice that seemed to be coming from another room. My wife might live only a few months.

I told myself that I needed to focus on what the doctor was about to say rather than what she had just said. I thought to myself, *Look at the doctor and that will help you keep your composure*. I really needed to grasp the details of what she was saying.

The doctor did offer a small glimmer of hope. If we could shrink the tumor and it was not imbedded in the chest wall, then maybe it could be removed. She told us about Dr. Denise Yardley, one of the finest oncologists in the southeast. She had a successful track record of shrinking similar tumors. A round of chemotherapy might shrink the tumor enough for surgery. Dr. Dunbar was a personal friend of Dr. Yardley. She promised to try to arrange an appointment for us with the highly sought after specialist.

The ride home was one of both quiet talk and reflection. Now we at least knew what we were up against. The fear of the unknown was out of the way. As we rode along, we talked about what we had just heard.

Diana confided in me her hope of cure and full recovery. Deep down in my heart, I was just not sure. I knew God was in control, but I did not know how to feel. I wanted to attack the cancer with every means at our disposal. I wish I could have felt one hundred percent that she was going to beat this. I believed in God's ability to heal, and I had seen a number of folks who were cancer survivors. Would Diana be one of these? I had such an unsettled feeling. My prayers were for her cure and full recovery. I did not want to think otherwise. Again, I had to trust God and believe he would do what was best.

The appointment with Dr. Yardley was secured, and we felt so excited to have one of the best oncologists in our state on our team. In one sense, it was encouraging because we were about to begin the journey down the road to recovery. On the other hand, we were stepping into a world that was new and strange to us.

We were willing to take that step. Even though we were "sailing into uncharted waters," we had great confidence in God above. We had placed everything in his hands. We had made him captain of our lives many years ago. We were not sure what lay ahead, but he had proven throughout the journey of our lives up to this point that he was very capable of bringing us into the safe haven of his harbor.

I will never forget the first visit a week later to Dr. Yardley's office. Although I had visited several cancer patients in hospital rooms and homes in my role as a pastor, I had no idea how many people this horrible disease affected.

This is true of many caregivers. The fact is there are diseases out there that affect so many people and require time and attention of caregivers. Cancer is only one. ALS (Lou Gehrig's disease), Alzheimer's, multiple sclerosis, stroke, crippling arthritis, muscular dystrophy, cerebral palsy, spinal bi da and severe mental retardation to name a few on a long list of people who need help from a loving caregiver.

Every situation is different, but each requires a devoted loved one or friend who sacrificially gives his or her time, talent, and treasures to provide that personal care. Doctors' offices and treatment facilities are crowded and over owing with those trapped by a disease and situation not of their own making.

The waiting area was filled with patients and their families. Patients treated in this facility ranged from late teens to the nineties. A few waited alone, but most had the support of a family member or friend. It felt a little strange as we approached the receptionist. Diana introduced herself and handed the lady at the desk a large manila envelope with paperwork from Dr. Dunbar's office. They photocopied our insurance card, and we quietly made our way to a couple of empty seats near the back of the room. The amount of paperwork necessary for initial examinations, referrals, and treatment is a necessary evil. If you are a caregiver, more is always better. Take everything you think you might need and a few things you might not need.

One thing that struck me as a little funny were the number of people glued to the TV set. It was tuned to a local channel, and soap operas seemed to be the popular shows of the day. I thought to myself, *I haven't seen a soap opera since I was a boy at home when my mother was a big fan.* No, I didn't get hooked as a result.

We sat for almost an hour before we were called to the lab, where Diana was weighed and her blood drawn. Then we stepped into a small examination room. The visit to the lab and being ushered to small examination rooms would become a regular routine for the next three years. The room was typical of most doctors' office examination rooms. I did notice one difference from others that I had seen. It had on dis- play a variety of wall diagrams and literature on cancer and breast cancer in particular. It brought home the sense of where we were and why we were there.

Dr. Yardley, a professional-looking woman in her mid forties, entered the room and introduced herself. She used one of those wall diagrams to illustrate the particular type cancer Diana had and how it was progressing. She followed her explanation with a pro- posed four-step treatment plan.

1. A combination of drugs in six massive doses would be administered over an eighteen-week period. The dosage required a five- to six-hour treatment once every three weeks.

2. If chemotherapy was successful, a surgeon would perform a radical mastectomy, removing the cancerous left breast.

3. Thirty- five radiation treatments would follow the surgery, one each day, five days a week for seven weeks.

4. Diana could expect to take chemotherapy orally for the rest of her life.

It is so important to develop a plan for treatment. Dr. Yardley methodically described the proposed plan for Diana's treatment. The whole process would begin with minor surgery to implant an object called a port. A port describes the function of the object, an access point for the infusion of chemicals directly into the bloodstream. The port would be placed under the skin just below the neckline so it could be hidden underneath Diana's clothing.

The implanting of a port, we learned later on, was a very common practice for cancer patients requiring chemotherapy. We were a little concerned about the port being implanted to begin with, but learned that it would make it much easier on Diana in the long run. When Diana actually began her treatments, we were so glad that the port had been put in. It did save her arms from what would have been a great deal of pain from numerous puncture wounds caused by a multitude of needles and injections. The port was a good thing, I would highly recommend it.

Dr. Yardley knew we would probably have concerns and questions about the proposed plan of treatment she had just prescribed, she opened it up for us to ask any questions we might have. Diana asked,

"What are possible side effects of the suggested chemotherapy treatment?"

The answer was horrifying. Doctor Yardley said, "You will probably lose your hair. You may get open sores in your mouth. You may become nauseated with vomiting and diarrhea. Your resistance to infection and disease will be lowered. You may need an occasional special shot to elevate your blood count. You will feel weak at times and suffer bouts of fatigue. You may suffer some depression and mood swings. Your taste buds may be affected."

We really could not fully comprehend the magnitude of the side effects being suggested. We talked about them on the way home. Diana expressed how she hoped she would not lose her hair. She had the most beautiful, dark black hair. Her mother was part Cherokee Indian, and her dark hair really complimented her pearl white skin and bright blue eyes. She reminded me that not everyone lost their hair with chemotherapy treatments. "Maybe I'll be one of the lucky ones and be able to keep mine," she said with a hopeful sound in her voice. I agreed that certainly that was a possibility and maybe she wouldn't. We both were hoping. I could not imagine her any other way.

When asked where the treatments would be administered, we learned that most oncology centers had treatment facilities on site. Tennessee Oncology, where doctor Yardley's office was located, had excellent treatment facilities. Later that afternoon we were taken on a tour of the treatment facility and introduced to the staff. It was equipped with a large treatment room with several treatment stations. The room was furnished with a variety of resources to make the experience as comfortable as possible. These included recliners, televisions with earphones, and light snacks.

Doctor Yardley explained how things would proceed in the treatment room. While Diana relaxed in a recliner, a nurse would bring the prescribed chemicals to her and use the new port to insert the medication directly into the bloodstream. While receiving her treatments, she could nap, read, watch TV, talk with me, pray, or whatever she cared to do. The chemotherapy IV was placed on a portable caddy. Diana would be able to get up, walk around, and go to the restroom. She would have freedom of movement while receiving treatment. She simply had to roll the caddy around with her. Treatments often lasted up to six hours.

Diana's questions continued. "Will taking these

drugs really shrink the tumor enough for the surgery to be performed?"

"We've had great success in shrinking tumors in other patients, but each tumor is different. However, I feel really good about your chances." She told us that we would receive more information about surgery from Dr. Dunbar when the procedure became possible.

She went on to answer our questions about radiation therapy. *Why take the radiation? Will it hurt? Does it burn? How long does it last?*

She explained that radiation therapy had been greatly improved. Diana would not feel anything. The treatments would not burn. Each application would last only a few seconds and would be administered to several locations in the chest area. She did warn that radiation often left patients feeling tired but recommended the treatments as a preventive measure to kill any cancerous cells remaining after surgery.

She explained that treatment was only the beginning. After the radiation, Diana would be tested regularly and treated accordingly.

When Diana asked the inevitable question—
"Will I ever be cancer free?"—the doctor responded,
"No one can predict the future, but if we can get you
to the five-year mark, you have a good chance of
living a long life."

As we left the doctor's office that day, we still
had many questions. As we drove down the road on
our way home, we talked about what we had just
heard a few minutes earlier. Many encouraging
things had happened. We now had a definite sense of
direction. We had agreed to a treatment plan of
action. Five years seemed so far in the future, but
maybe, just maybe we could reach that milestone.

Even though we had launched out into waters
uncharted to us, we had great trust in the captain of
our ship. No waters were uncharted to him. We
trusted him to guide us through the storm we were
experiencing and to bring us safely to the other side
into his safe haven. Now we even had a goal to strive
for.

Caregiver Principles

- Leave the safety of the shoreline of your own
  thinking and launch into the depths of God's
  marvelous care.

- Develop a treatment plan of action and set the wheels of that plan into motion.

- Hold tightly to each other's hands as you sail together into those dark uncharted waters, which may lie just ahead.

- Make a conscious decision to let God be the captain of the ship of your lives.

- Have faith in God and trust him to guide you through these difficult days and to bring you into his safe harbor.

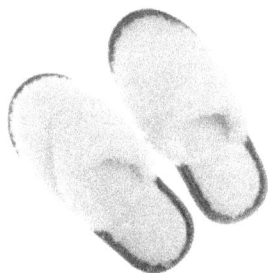

experiencing
the unbelievable

As we waited for therapy to start, days turned into
weeks. Those weeks of waiting were some of the
hard- est. The time seemed to pass so slowly. We
continued our regular schedules as best we could, but
the disease was not far from our thinking. I could not
understand why it took so long to begin the
treatments. Surely the tumor was growing larger and
more difficult to treat with each passing day. I
learned that waiting was standard practice, not
because medical personnel lacked concern but
because huge numbers of people are diagnosed with
cancer each day.

If you are in the beginning stages of providing care for a relative or close friend, try not to get discouraged with the delays in treatment that often occur. It is normal in most cases.

Three weeks passed, and finally the day arrived for treatment to begin. We drove the twenty or so miles from our house to the treatment facility near downtown. We parked across the street and walked in with a sense of anticipation. We were about to begin. We checked in at the front desk and soon heard Diana's name called by a nurse. We followed the nurse to the lab and then on to the second waiting room on the right.

A nurse weighed Diana, pricked her finger to test her blood count, and drew two vials of blood for map- ping and further testing. We repeated this same routine at each of more than one hundred visits at this office and a variety of other facilities. We were excited as we prepared to move forward.

We followed the nurse into the small six-by-ten foot examining room with no windows. We waited to be called to the large treatment room. After waiting for what seemed an eternity, Diana received additional x-rays to determine if the tumor had changed. I sensed something was not right. *Has the cancer gotten worse? Is the treatment room full? Do we have to wait for someone to leave?* Surely they wouldn't postpone the treatment after all the days of waiting and mental preparation. They wouldn't dare crush our emotions by making us leave without a treatment!

When Dr. Yardley entered the room, she had a serious look on her face and a large envelope in her hand. A new spot had appeared on the x-ray in addition to the tumor. The tumor was in the left breast, but this spot was in the right lung. She told us the spot was a pocket of fluid that would have to be removed. To make matters worse, chemotherapy could not begin until the procedure was completed.

Hearing the news felt like someone had made a fist and hit both Diana and me in the stomach. Diana immediately asked, "What caused the fluid? Could the cancer have caused it?" Up to this point, we all, including the doctors, thought the cancer was contained in one breast. If the fluid contained diseased cells, then the cancer had spread and could be any- where in her body.

Dr. Yardley described the process of removing the fluid through a procedure called a thorosynthesis. My heart ached as she told how a large syringe with a long needle would be pushed into Diana's back through the muscles of her ribcage into the back part of her lung. She would have to remain awake and alert, so there would be no anesthetic. She would feel that sharp needle force its way through her skin, muscles, ribcage, and into her right lung. The pocket of fluid would then be drawn from the lung with the syringe.

I fought back tears as the doctor explained what she could expect. I struggled to keep my composure. We had not even left the starting blocks, yet we were back to square one. I felt a ash of anger for a moment. This was so unfair to Diana. The cancer was bad enough for her to deal with, and now, she had to face something like this.

Even worse, we had been so up *emotionally* to begin the chemotherapy, and now that would be postponed and who knew for how long. I kept quiet and I'm glad I did. Sometimes the better part of valor is to bite your tongue. If you are a caregiver, please remember that emotions come and go. You can't control how you feel, but you must control what you do with those feelings. You will feel anger and disappointment at times. It's *okay* to have those feelings. Try to stop and think a moment before you put feelings into words. Sometimes a few minutes of thought will help you react in a way that will produce a much better result.

When Dr. Yardley asked Diana how quickly she wanted to have the procedure done, she replied, "As soon as possible!" A nurse made some calls to see how soon the thorosynthesis could be arranged. After another long wait, the doctor and nurse returned. It was twelve thirty p.m. If we could make the cross-town trip to St. Thomas Hospital by one, the procedure could be done immediately. Diana's first chemotherapy treatment could be rescheduled for the following week.

After speeding through town, we arrived at St. Thomas with only ten minutes to spare. As we walked across the parking lot, Diana's knees buckled and she began to weep. The recent turn of events was almost more than she could bear. Placing my arm around her waist, helping her walk, I assured her everything would be okay. She regained her composure and I held her hand as we walked in to face this sad and painful ordeal together.

Another waiting room, another check in desk, another ordeal of waiting, this process would repeat itself many times over the coming years. I felt helpless sitting alone while Diana was led through a door and back to parts of the hospital unknown to either of us. I could only imagine the ordeal of pain and suffering she was undergoing through this most difficult procedure. I sat quietly trying to browse out-of-date magazines and half heartedly listening to the TV in the small waiting area. People came and went and time slowly passed. Finally, a male nurse called the name "Mr. Harris," and I rose from my chair with an uneasy feeling as I walked through a door and passed a number of patients who each were there for outpatient treatments.

I made a right turn and found Diana on a treatment bed laying on her left side. I immediately tried to read her countenance to see how she was doing. She was in obvious pain. She had to lay there for another hour or so to make sure the wound created by the long needle closed properly. Also, as a precaution, they were keeping close watch on the right lung. There is always the possibility of collapsing a lung when a lung is punctured either by accident or through a medical procedure.

We finally were ready to drive home. I pulled the car near the entry door to the hospital, and they brought Diana out in a wheel chair. She was really tired but wanted to share the entire procedure details with me. She needed to talk and I wanted her to. I quietly drove the approximately thirty miles home as she went through each step of the procedure.

My emotions swelled within me as I wished some- how I could have taken her place and had the procedure done to me instead of her. The procedure came alive in my own mind as she described the pain of the needle moving its way through her skin, muscle, back, ribcage, chest cavity, and finally the back side of her lung. I could feel my eyes watering not able to imagine how painful this must have been without anesthesia.

A week later, the terrible pain of the previous week had subsided. Surely Diana was about to finally begin her road to her recovery. Maybe cancer was only a bump in the road for us and life would soon return to normal. We returned to the same small examining room and waited for Dr. Yardley.

The expression on her face as she entered the room indicated something serious was in store for us. After earlier telling us the first of eighteen weeks of chemo- therapy would begin that day, she paused. Then, with regret in her voice, she said, "I'm sorry to have to tell you this, but we found cancer cells in the fluid sample taken from your right lung. This means the cancer is not contained and has spread." A rush of anxiety came over me. My anxiety centered on knowing something had changed but not knowing the magnitude of what her words meant.

When we asked her to explain what this meant, she told us cancer cells could show up anywhere in Diana's body and at any time. She further stated that Diana would probably never be completely cancer free. She did offer hope that the ravenous disease might be held in check.

We could not fully understand what all that meant at that moment. I do remember talking on the way home after the treatment about what Dr. Yardley had said. I thought that just as the cancer cells had moved outside the breast, my logic told me that the chemo   therapy would also reach throughout the body. Maybe the treatment would work, and the cancer would be attacked and arrested.

Chemotherapy

Finally, after four weeks of anxious waiting, treatment began. We both listened intently as the nurse explained the mix of drugs that would be injected into Diana's system. One was ruby red in color, the other clear. I found myself uneasy as I watched the poison designed to shrink the tumor and kill the cancer cells move slowly from the IV, through the port, and into her blood stream.

Even though I felt uneasy, I also felt a sense of relief. It was as though I had a release emotionally. We had waited so long, but now something was finally happening.

At last we had something to fight the disease attacking her body. However, after years of visiting people in the hospital as a pastor, I knew that one side effect of chemotherapy was that it killed good cells along with the cancerous cells. I knew that for the foreseeable future Diana would not be the same.

I wondered in my mind how things might change. Would this affect her personality? I knew that it would probably impact her physically. I loved her for who she was not just how she looked, so I knew I could handle those changes. I worried a little about the personality and emotional changes. Would she become more dependent on me? Would she continue to be the kind, tender lady I had fallen in love with and married? Would our relationship change as a result of this cancer and chemotherapy? I would find answers to those questions and others over the next few years of the illness.

The hours passed slowly. I sat quietly beside my wife as she drifted off to sleep. This first treatment was the beginning of a process that would be repeated every three weeks throughout the entire summer.

We came home, and supper was waiting. Diana seemed to be doing ne, yet when we sat down to eat she became nauseatcd and rushed to the restroom. I felt a pain in the middle of my gut. I ached for her as she lost her supper in the restroom. What could I do to help I thought to myself? I dampened a washcloth with warm water, washed her face, and led her to our bedroom. I laid the cloth on her forehead and she drifted off to sleep. The side effects of chemotherapy had begun.

If you are a caregiver, it is not so important what you do, but that you are close by and there. Your loved one or friend needs to know that someone is close by and can assist if needed. It will be the little things you do that will make the difference for them.

The side effects would show up in a variety of ways. About two weeks after the first treatment, when Diana was getting dressed for the day, she suddenly called my name. Hearing the anxiety in her voice, I looked up to see her pull a handful of her beautiful black hair from her head.

We knew that this possible side effect was a probability, but when it arrived it still came as a shock. As a caregiver, many such abrupt incidents may arise. How you react can have profound and long-term effects. I had previously thought about how I might react ahead of time if this happened. I had recited to myself what I might say. Now, here it was. I'm so glad I anticipated this possibility.

I reminded her that I loved her and let her cry on my shoulder. I told her we would take care of it that night. I called her sister Dorene and my daughter Missy and told them what happened. Missy came over that night and shaved Diana's head, replacing her natural hair with one of the wigs selected ahead of time.

Selecting the wigs, scarves, etc., ahead of time really helped make the side effect more bearable. If you can anticipate and prepare for things that the doctors and others who had similar experiences share with you, it may help the situation be much more bearable.

As treatments continued, I tried to protect Diana's privacy. Even though her appearance had changed and she had lost her hair, it did not matter to me. She was afraid of how I might react if I saw her completely bald. I never entered the bedroom or bathroom with- out knocking first and receiving her permission.

This awkward pattern for husband and wife continued from mid-May until the week of Independence Day. Then the inevitable happened. During our annual Gatlinburg vacation with most of Diana's side of the family, I thought Diana, Dorene, and the girls had gone shopping. To my surprise, when I entered the back bedroom to retrieve some notes to finish preparing a sermon, Diana was changing clothes. She did not have on her wig.

I thought I was prepared for that moment. I had anticipated it and talked through it to myself two or three times. I could not help myself. I stopped dead in my tracks. I thought to myself, *Should I say excuse me and leave the room? Should I say something complimentary? What should I do?*

She was completely bald. It was the rst time I had seen her that way. I will always remember the look on her face. Her look told me she felt unattractive and unsure of herself. I knew my reaction and what I said at that moment would have a long-term effect on her and our relationship. Her eyes locked with mine. I met her gaze and forced myself not to look at her head. I quickly embraced her and told her how much I loved her, that it did not make any difference at all to me. I had always been totally honest with her, and she knew I meant what I said.

I did learn something valuable through what we had just experienced. Timing is so important in every relationship. Respect for privacy is also important. As a caregiver, it's important not to assume or rush some things. Allowing your loved one or friend the dignity of privacy is paramount. Let privacy reign supreme and let them share things of an intimate nature at the time of their choosing.

I'm glad I afforded her that privacy. Even though we experienced a moment of awkwardness, I left the room feeling that, for the last three months, I had tried my best to do the right thing. A large part of care giving is simply trying your best to do the right thing. That can take different forms depending on the situation. It should always be done in a way that extends respect, compassion, and dignity to the person you are caring for. If and when your role as a caregiver comes to an end and you look back and can say, *I always tried to do the right thing*, it will help you feel good about yourself and how you cared for your loved one or friend.

When the chemotherapy treatments were finally completed, the doctors told us the treatment had been a success. The tumor had been reduced dramatically. It appeared not to be imbedded in the chest wall, and the surgery could be attempted.

This was a great day for us. This opened the door for the other treatment steps earlier outlined by Dr. Yardley. One cannot comprehend what a sense of relief and excitement this news brought to me, Diana, our children, our extended family, church family, and friends. We had so many people across the nation who had prayed for this result. We felt that God was listening and answering our prayers.

The side effects were no fun but worth the end result. We were anxious to move on to the second step of the treatment plan.

Surgery

Developing confidence in one's doctor is important. We were headed back to the kind and caring Dr. Dunbar. She too was excited to hear the news of the successful first step from Dr. Yardley. We received the call from her office informing us of the time and place where the surgery would be performed. I remember feeling really good about the progress we were seeing in the treatment of Diana's disease. The ball seemed to be really rolling now.

Diana and I both felt upbeat and encouraged. The slow start had given way to a gradual increase in the process. If we could just get the tumor out of her body, things were bound to be better for her. We had attacked it with the chemotherapy and now were going to remove it from its source of nourishment and kill it. We were both ready.

On the appointed day, we checked into Baptist Hospital, prayed together, and she was taken away to surgery. Another chapter in the life-and-death struggle to save her life was about to begin.

The children, Doreen and I along with many friends made our way to the surgery waiting area, a place that would become very familiar to me over the next few years. The hours passed quickly; the surgery actually took less time than expected.

Dr. Dunbar delivered the report in person. The news was good. The tumor was not embedded in the chest wall, and they were able to get all of it. Diana would only remain in the hospital a few days.

The sense of relief was unbelievable. The tumor was gone. The thing that had created so many problems was out. They were able to get it all. It was not attached to the chest wall. I thought to myself that the report could not have been any better. I thanked God for answering our prayers. That was another one of those "good days" we experienced during Diana's illness.

The family and I made our way to her room. I spent the night by her side, introducing myself to the recliner next to her bed. Over time, that chair became an old and familiar friend to me.

Unless you've experienced *nightlife* in the hospital by the bed of a loved one or friend, it's hard to under- stand how uncomfortable it can be. Sleep is confined to short intervals due to the needed interruptions by hospital staff to care for their patients. One will be restless, constantly watching and listening and attempting to be attentive to the needs of that loved one or friend. The restless night is long and leaves one tired and many times exhausted the next day. It is important to let others help by sparing you a night or two if the hospital stay is an extended one.

With the help of the medical team, Diana was able to get up and move around the next day. After a couple of days, they allowed her to shower. She refused the nurse's help and asked me to assist her. As she undressed, her face reflected the shame she felt. She felt less of a woman because of the surgery. "Will you look at me? I'm a freak!" Her words seemed to hang in midair as the reality of the surgery became obvious to us both.

With my heart breaking, I tenderly scolded her and told her she was not a freak, that she should never use those words again.

It was important for me not to look shocked or upset at her loss. My reaction and reassurance helped her accept herself as she was now instead of dwelling a long time on how she used to look. She grew to accept her body, and we both felt at ease quickly with the physical change she had undergone. I believe my attitude and acceptance played a huge role in her embracing the changes and moving on.

If your mate, other family member, or friend is impacted physically by an illness or surgery, please remember that they need acceptance and reassurance. They feel less a person and need to feel normal again. Your attitude can make such a difference.

Radiation

Diana healed from her surgery with no infection or complications, and we moved on to part three of the treatment plan—radiation therapy. We were pleased to reach this point. Two of the major parts of the plan had been completed. Two down and two to go, and the treatment plan would be completed.

This part would be less invasive physically for Diana. We learned through the experience of the treatment that it would have a lesser impact on her and my work schedules. We could go about our daily routines much as we had before Diana had been diagnosed with the disease. We anxiously awaited the day when radiation therapy would begin.

We arrived at the Medical Plaza building and rode the elevator below ground to the radiation treatment area. After filling out the necessary paperwork, we waited our turn.

Diana's first treatment took less than ten minutes. We returned another thirty-four times during the next seven weeks to complete the number of treatments ordered by the oncologist. The treatments were not painful. The only side effect we noticed was fatigue.

Diana seemed to tire more easily as we neared the final week of treatments.

If your care giving circumstances permit the person receiving care to continue to work or stay at home by themselves, you may want to consider an early morning appointment. Many radiation treatment facilities begin treatments at seven-thirty in the morning. We were able to secure the seven-thirty appointment slot and were both able to be at work by eight-thirty. If you are able to be home with your loved one or friend, an early appointment can free you up for other things during the day. Remember, most radiation treatments are from ten to thirty- five treatments over a period of weeks.

We thought, after completing the chemotherapy and radiation, that finally the ordeal was nearing its end and life was about to return to normal.

I learned some valuable lessons during those eight months. I learned real love transcends the physical. I watched Diana's attitude change through the terrible days of chemotherapy.

Women care deeply about their appearances. I saw her accept the loss of part of her womanhood and move on. Each day she drew closer to the Lord. I never heard her complain or get angry at God. She continued to be faithful in her prayer life and daily devotions. I watched her attend church, except for a few times when the treatments left her too weak and sick to do so.

Caregiver Principles

- You must try and remain strong for the sake of your mate and children.

- Try and put into practice those biblical principles you have learned.

- Believe that God is real.

- Believe that God is always present.

- Believe that God knows and loves you.

- Believe God can be trusted with your life and the lives of those you care about.

- Remember that God is a guiding light through your darkest hours.

when your world seems to be turning right side up

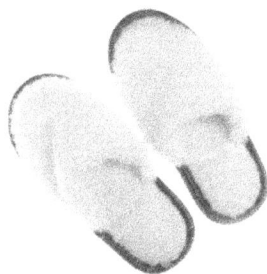

Finally, we received something good from the doctor. We moved to the best year of the disease. The harsh treatments were over, and things were returning to a somewhat normal state. God had blessed us with a third grandchild in the midst of the chemotherapy treatments. Diana referred to "Claire Bear" as God's special gift to her in the midst of a terrible time in her life.

Our family had grown to nine, and when they all came together in our home, it became pretty crowded. We determined we really needed more room. For the past couple of years we had talked about the possibility of finding another home in the suburbs of Nashville.

I decided that building a new home might be just the distraction Diana needed to go on with her life. She showed great interest in the idea.

We looked at several existing homes but did not find the one that seemed right for us. We located a nice subdivision only a few miles from Diana's work place with a few building lots still available. We selected a lot and began working on plans together and were able to build a new home. The details of decorating and the time of looking forward to the move were a great help to Diana. The home was finished, and we moved in. It was an exciting time.

Things were going well at the church I pastored in Nashville, Tennessee. The kids and grandkids were all doing well. We just knew the worst was over and things were about to get back to normal. The second year was off to a great start.

Even though we continued with regular visits to the oncologist, the reports were good. We enjoyed those days. It seemed like our upside-down world was righting itself.

We did not realize it at the time, but these would be the most stress free and relaxing days of the disease. It was as if God placed a time of rest in our lives to help us regain our physical and emotional strength.

No matter how difficult the circumstances seem that one might be experiencing, wonderful lessons can be learned from God during that period of time.

Caregiver Principles

- God sometimes places a pause in between difficult days to help you catch your breath, regain strength, and restore hope for the future.

- Learn to enjoy life and live it one day at a time.

- Remember that you can't live in the past, and the future doesn't exist.

- Trust the Scriptures, which remind us not to worry about tomorrow because tomorrow will take care of itself.

- Enjoy the moments you have with that loved one or friend.

- Celebrate good news and give praise to the Lord for his goodness.

- Take a few moments to reflect on all your blessings and see what God has done for you and your family.

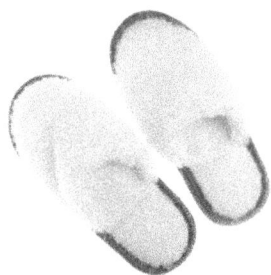

this can't be happening again!

It was hard to believe two years had passed since we had received the news of Diana's cancer. The second year had been a good one, although I had noticed Diana was tiring much more quickly toward the close of the year. She was on a morphine patch because of the pain she had begun experiencing. It left her drowsy at times, and she went to bed almost as soon as she arrived home from work. She wanted to continue working. I agreed only because I felt it gave her a sense of purpose and something to look forward to each day.

I could tell she was not improving. I did not want to admit to myself that she was beginning to decline. Events sometimes have a way of coldly thrusting reality upon us.

During the darkest part of the night, I awoke to a sharp kick to the back of my right leg. As I struggled to open my eyes, I knew that something was terribly wrong.

I sat up in bed and realized that Diana was out of control, jerking violently. Her legs were moving in a kicking motion. Her head was thrown back, and she was semiconscious. She couldn't tell me what was wrong. She couldn't control her arms. I didn't know what to do. I had never seen a look like I saw on her face.

My heart raced. I was so scared. I honestly thought she was dying, and I didn't know what to do. I knew if I waited on an ambulance she might die before they arrived and got her to a hospital.

I quickly threw on some clothes, wrapped Diana in something, and carried her to the car. She continued to be physically out of control. I raced to the new hospital that had just opened a mile from our house.

When we arrived at the emergency entrance, I ran in and told them I thought my wife was dying. A whole crew of doctors and nurses ran out to the car with me. Little did we know this would be the first of many such trips to emergency rooms.

The emergency room doctor examined Diana and determined that she was experiencing a seizure. He ordered a shot, and the seizure subsided. He asked about her medical history, and I gave him a rundown. He wanted to call in a neurologist to help determine the cause of the seizures. I agreed, but I knew the hospital we were in was not on our insurance plan. The next couple of days were traumatic. The seizures continued. The doctors were afraid the cancer had spread to Diana's brain.

I remember that during the second day a bean counter from accounting came up to our room. I could not believe she would want to talk of such things in front of the patient. She informed me in front of Diana that insurance would not cover another day in their hospital. I would have to be personally responsible for the bill.

I couldn't believe what I was hearing. Even worse, Diana was hearing it also. She began to cry, and I became angry. I asked the lady to step into the hall- way. I told her we did not even know what was causing these seizures. We had to keep her there until we determined the best course of treatment. If that meant I must be responsible for the bill, then so be it.

In the end, I had to pay almost $4,000 out of pocket for that extra day in the hospital.

After several tests, we determined the lining of Diana's brain had been damaged by the chemotherapy and she would probably experience many more such episodes. They tried a variety of medications and finally provided one that helped.

The seizures continued for another nine months. They finally slowed and could be kept under control with medication. The medication had to be taken on time, or a seizure would occur. I also had a special medication that could be given at the first sign of an impending seizure.

I would awake in the middle of the night at Diana's slightest movement and pay close attention to deter- mine if a seizure was coming. I would then be awake for hours because of the adrenalin rush I had experienced. It would be almost two years before I could rest easy enough to sleep most of the night.

How does one cope when hope is dashed? In those dark nights when it was so quiet and I felt so alone, I reminded myself over and over again that God was there. I knew that I was the only link between arresting a seizure quickly and Diana violently careening physically out of control. I so needed God's help. He was the only one who could help me, and he did, time after time.

So many times with tears in my eyes I would quietly cry out to him. I would feel the tender touch of his Spirit and a sense that it would be all right. I am not one who shows much emotion—period. During those dark nights, I looked to God for help. I found that it helped me to raise a hand toward heaven with my head bowed and reach for his touch. I would feel his touch, and his presence would help the darkness to pass. The sun would finally break through the window, and we had made it through another night. Truly God is good, and every promise of his word is true and is just as available today as it was in past generations.

Caregiver Principles

- Remind yourself that God is really still there.

- God will help you in the midst of the darkest hour of the night when no one else can.

- He understands your need for a tender touch and a kind word. Cry out to him and maybe shed a tear.

- Great reassurance can come from raising

your right hand toward heaven and asking God to
touch you and take you by the hand.

- He will give you a special peace that only comes
  in the midst of life's most violent storms.

- Look to him. Look for him.

- The night will pass. The morning will come. You
  will make it through.

- "For the Lord is good; his mercy is everlasting;
  and his truth endures to all generations" (Psalm
  100:5 nkjv).

taking care of yourself

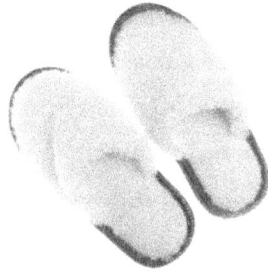

One of the hardest things to think about while caring for a terminally ill loved one is oneself. One becomes so focused on giving time and attention to another that he can easily forget how important it is to take care of his own mind and body. The stress of giving care can and will weigh heavily on one's mental and physical well being. Dealing with mental stress is an absolute must if one is to keep balance and provide the best personal care possible.

Finding an outlet or diversion from the illness is an absolute must if one is to find personal balance and remain emotionally healthy. The diversion can be most anything, but it should involve being away from the house and ill loved one for varying periods of time. I well remember the day my brother-in-law asked me if I wanted to take his Honda scooter for a spin. It had been years since I had ridden a motorcycle.

I was a little nervous when I sat down on it. I owned a motorcycle in my early twenties, but now I was about to turn fifty. I certainly didn't want to embarrass myself, to say nothing of wrecking Sam's motorcycle. I took a deep breath and gave it a try.

My nervousness left me quickly, and I thoroughly enjoyed the ride. I mentioned it to Diana, and she sensed a spark of excitement that hadn't been there for many months. There was something special about being in the openness of the outdoors that had taken my mind off the terrible disease and ordeal we were going through. I had something to focus on that I enjoyed.

Before long, Diana encouraged me to look into buying a used one. I finally settled on a Harley-Davidson Sportster. I ended up buying a new 2003 model in the fall of 2004. I had found my outlet. I began a pattern that continues until this day. I would get out by myself on the motorcycle for thirty minutes to an hour at a time.

Sometimes I would trailer the bike over to my sister-in-law's home in Cookeville, Tennessee, about an hour and a half away. Diana would spend time with her sister Dorene while Sam and I spent hours riding in the mountains. I would be away from my role for a few hours and return refreshed, rejuvenated, and ready to carry on.

After Diana's death and at the urging of my children, I bought an even larger motorcycle and spent many hours alone riding. I was able to talk to the Lord, think about life, and work my way through the grief.

No, I am not suggesting everyone should rush out and purchase a motorcycle. I am suggesting each per- son should find something he or she enjoys doing that provides a short diversion from the caregiving role.

Looking after one's physical health is also important. Regular exercise and good eating habits are essential if one is to be at his best. The stress of giving care can take a horrendous physical toll. Junk food and unhealthy snacks can become substitutes for balanced healthy meals. Especially as the disease progresses, much time is spent in hospital rooms and/or sitting at home with the loved one.

Added pounds will appear. Energy levels drop. Blood pressure can rise. If one is not careful, he will injure his own health and become a burden instead of a help. It is important to think about what one is eating. Stepping on the bathroom scales can be a shock but also provides regular reminders of how one is doing on the health front.

What about exercise? Who has time when you are preparing meals, cleaning house, washing clothes, and making numerous medical visits to doctors' offices, hospitals, and laboratories? Exercise is so important.

A membership at the YMCA or a health club can be the stimulus that prompts one to make time to exercise. Making a financial investment is usually enough to provide motivation for one to get her money's worth. Getting away for an hour or so three times a week can work wonders.

Swimming is a great exercise. It is easy on the joints, tones the muscles, and strengthens the heart and lungs. It also helps keep the weight down. One might be amazed at how well his health can be impacted in a positive way with consistent exercise.

I am not saying one should run out and join the nearest health club and start swimming tomorrow. Other forms of exercise can be effective and enjoy-able. Walking is a good way to stay healthy and t. Most indoor shopping malls are happy for walkers to use their facilities, especially before the stores open in the morning. If one attempts to walk outside, he will find days that are not suitable for walking. Rain, snow, winter cold, and summer heat can be serious obstacles to walking outside. Joining the YMCA or a local health club can provide opportunities for other exercise-related activities as well.

Find something you enjoy doing to distract you from all you are dealing with at home. You will not be deserting or neglecting your loved ones. It will be good for them to be away from you once in a while. That will help them mentally.

Many times they feel they are dominating too much of your time. They feel like a burden. They feel they are keeping you from doing things you enjoy and would like to do. They feel guilty. When they see you taking care of yourself physically and emotionally, it makes them feel better about the whole situation. When you do something just because you enjoy it, it makes them happy.

Caregiver Principles

• Think about one thing that comes to mind right now that you enjoy doing and haven't done in a while and seriously consider if it might be the diversion you need.

- Take a serious look at your eating habits.

- Develop a consistent plan for regular exercise.

- Find ways to relieve stress and sharpen the mind.

- Try and put a smile on your face and watch how it encourages you and others around you.

- You'll be much more effective at giving care to your loved one if you are mentally and physically healthy and strong.

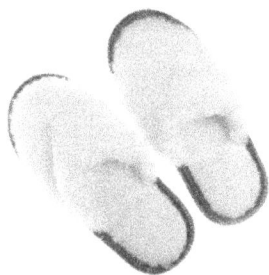

help! i need somebody!

Giving care to a dying loved one is a twenty-four-hour, seven-day-a-week job. Our tendency is to try and become Superman or Superwoman and handle it alone. It seems like an imposition to let others help. After all, they have families and problems of their own.

Letting others help is hard to do. Probably at some point one will not have a choice. I remember thinking that this was my wife and no one could look after her as well as I could. It was my responsibility, and I would handle it. I have a news ash for you. Superman and Superwoman did really well most of the time, but they even had problems they could not handle alone.

You will do well for a while. But the time will come when you will get worn down little by little. You will find yourself physically and emotionally drained. You will need others to step in and give you relief.

I would encourage you to accept help earlier rather than later. It is so important for you to maintain your physical and emotional strength.

Who are these others, and how can they help? Family members can be the greatest source of help. There will normally be one person who wants to help, is capable, and has the time.

We had such a person. Diana's younger sister. Dorene became a lifesaver for me. She loved her sister and was willing to do whatever was necessary to help her. She not only said *if* you need anything let us know, she went one giant step further by seeking ways to help.

Maybe you are reading this book to better under- stand and help those who are primary caregivers to others. Extending an offer to help is a wonderful thing. Let me encourage you to go one step further. Find specific ways to help.

Dorene and her husband, Sam, made the hour-plus drive from their home to ours many times to help us. Dorene would relieve me by spending nights in the hospital room with Diana. She learned along with me how to drain fluid, change bandages, and give necessary medications. She helped Diana bathe and dress. She would come and spend a few days at a time helping with meals, laundry, doctor visits, and other things too numerous to mention.

There were a few times when I had gone just about as far as I could go and Dorene stepped in, sensing we needed someone to help us at that moment. I can never thank her enough and give her the praise she is due. I will never forget all that she and Sam did during numerous difficult periods of time.

There may be a Dorene in your family. Let that person help you. You need it now, or you will need it in the future.

You may be a *Dorene* yourself. God may impress you to help someone in your family or a friend who desperately needs relief. You can make a huge difference in someone's life. Go for it. Do more than offer. Inform your care giving family member or friend that you are going to do something particular for them. Do not be a bully but do mention something specific you wish to do for them. You may be amazed what a blessing it is to you and what tremendous help it is for the caregiver.

Another important area is your finances. Insurance helps, but there are many out-of-pocket expenses that cause money to become a real issue. I remember one difficult time we faced. Our savings were gone, and we owed a $3,000 hospital bill. I had already received a few ugly letters wanting payment. I had juggled bills and stayed current most of the way. I simply did not know what I was going to do.

I prayed about the need. God knew our struggle. He had been faithful in providing for us along the way. I went to the mailbox and found a handwritten note from my brother Rick and sister-in-law Ann. The note said, "We were thinking of you and thought maybe you could use this." A check for more than enough to cover the bill was with the note in the envelope. I stood in the driveway and wept.

My brother had worked hard, and God had blessed him financially. One reason I believe was because he was generous and maybe for such a time as this. He helped us more than once, wanting no praise or recognition. I will be eternally grateful, not only for the financial support, but for simply being there to encourage me during those difficult days.

Family and friends may want to help you *financially*. It will feel awkward, but God does move in mysterious ways. Do not keep someone from receiving a blessing God wants to give him or her. Let that person be blessed by God by giving to help you. That may be one of the ways God will provide for you.

Help may come from places you never imagined. I was pastor of one of the best churches in the world— Woodbine Free Will Baptist Church. Our church family stepped in and helped us in ways that were almost unbelievable. The church began by supplying our evening meal three days a week. Families signed up for specific days and would prepare and bring the meal to our home. Many times I would reheat left- overs the next day and one meal became two. This went on until I told them it was time to stop.

One great joy for us was to share a few moments with our church friends. They would bring the food by and many times help me get the meal ready. Sometimes only one person would come, many times the whole family. What a joy it was to have them in our home sharing the time of this illness with us. They felt they were in this thing with us. They felt a part of our lives, and I honestly believe it helped them feel closer to us and to pray with a more burdened heart for us. It also taught the valuable lesson of giving and God's wonderful love to many of their children.

This also did something very special for us. We were reminded that there were hundreds of people who loved us and thought of us often. It helped us not to feel alone even in the most difficult days.

They had special days for us. On one occasion the church took an offering to help us offset rising medical bills. The money amounted to thousands of dollars and reflected real sacrifice on the part of those good people. Ladies of the church would call and ask if they could come by and relieve me. They would order me to head out on my motorcycle or anything I would like to do to get away for a while.

I must mention one special lady. Norma was a lady in our church who loved my wife. She knew I was spending many hours per week giving care to Diana. She asked if she could talk with me. She said, "I feel that God is calling me to minister to Diana." She came by once a week, cleaned our house, and kept Diana company. She also asked if she could relieve me by taking Diana to some of the minor doctor checkups.

I called on Norma many times to help. I looked at all the visits to the doctor, lab work, hospital visits, special tests such as CAT scans and MRIs that we took Diana for in the last year of her life. There were over one hundred such visits. Norma helped me greatly during those days. I went to all the major visits, but Norma took Diana for a number of her regular visits. She helped me so much. I had church responsibilities that would have gone undone if it had not been for her.

Caregiver Principles

- If it's someone you trust and your loved one would feel safe with, take advantage of someone who offers to help you.

- We are often more blessed by helping others than receiving help from others. Allow someone else to be blessed by helping you and your loved one.

- Remember that people really do want to help. Give them an opportunity.

- Learn to graciously say *yes* and *thank you;* it can make your situation easier.

- Reach out and take that helping hand. You will be glad you did. God may be calling you to become a helping hand for those who desperately need one.

Why not pick out someone you can help? Find one or more specific things you can do to help. Make the offer to do those things for them. Extend that wonderful helping hand.

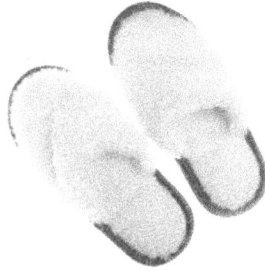

the descending shadow

Almost three years had passed since we first began the difficult journey. It had been obvious that Diana's future did not look good.

She was now confined to a wheel chair most of the time and on oxygen twenty-four hours a day. It was very difficult for Diana to walk up and down the steps to our second floor den due to her declining condition. We still were able to get out some, but it was always an ordeal. But at least she could get out of the house, and this was good for her mentally.

If you are a caregiver, there are options available with the confinement created by oxygen use. There is a machine that turns water into oxygen that can be rented for a small fee and makes things much easier. It comes complete with a forty-foot tube that permits the patient to move around the house fairly easily. Also, there are small portable tanks that can be rolled by the patient or hung on the back of a wheel chair that will permit you to make doctor visits, shop, grab a meal at a local restaurant, attend church services, etc. These tanks normally have a three-hour supply of oxygen. Always take a spare with you just in case you run low, and you will be amazed how much freedom this will afford for your loved one or friend as well as yourself.

Diana was offered a hospital bed to make it easier for her to get in and out of bed. I remember discussing it with her. She wanted to know if there was anything else we could do short of the hospital bed. I thought quickly, and I think the good Lord helped me. I offered the option of making a daytime bed on the couch in our living room just outside the master bedroom. It would be a comfortable place for her to rest, easily accessible for family and friends who came by and close to the half bathroom.

She indicated that was what she would like to do. We set up a small table next to the sofa for personal items she might need. I also brought one our small TVs from a bedroom into the living room, connected it to the cable outlet, and placed the remote on Diana's little table. She was very comfortable with this set up and made use of it for about three months. This worked out well for her and me also.

I remained home with her most of the time now.

My office was located upstairs, and I did not feel that I should be that far away from her. I needed internet access in order to do some of my work, so I set up a wireless system from my office and used my laptop downstairs near Diana. For almost three months I did most of my work sitting in the floor of our living room with my back against our loveseat less than ten feet from Diana.

She slept most of the time now. But I believe it gave her a sense of security to have me in the room and close to her. Many times I would look up from the computer to my left to see her eyes looking directly at me. Once in a while, I would give her a wink and many times a smile.

If you are a caregiver, maybe some of what I just mentioned may spark your thinking. One other thing that was helpful that you may want to consider.

Once I had Diana comfortable in the bed for the evening, I would spend a little time upstairs watching TV or simply trying to unwind from the stress of the day. I purchased two small hand held radios and placed one by her bedside and the other by my recliner upstairs. We used this to communicate just in case she needed me. This worked really well.

The fluid built up around her lungs had subsided, and doctors determined that the tube implanted months before was no longer necessary. The doctors felt it should be removed and the opening closed to reduce the possibility of infection. This would not be a difficult procedure but was a little risky because of her weakened physical condition.

The operation was scheduled for a few days later at Baptist Hospital. The surgery was performed and pronounced successful by the same surgeon who had implanted the tube earlier.

This was becoming almost a routine for us. So many procedures, so many hours in waiting before, during, and after surgeries, but this time would be drastically different. I was not ready for what I was about to hear.

The surgeon entered the waiting room, and I asked him how Diana was doing, meaning had she come through the surgery okay. Dorene was with us and heard my conversation with the doctor. His response caught me completely by surprise. He said, "She is not the same lady I saw a few months back when we implanted the drainage tube. She has declined drastically. Are you asking me how long she has to live?"

I was numb. I am not completely sure of the exact wording of the entire conversation. I mumbled, "Well, I guess so."

"She may have two months at the most."

His words seemed to hang in the air, a thick smothering haze. I would learn that his estimate was too optimistic. Of the many things I learned during this experience was that doctors do their best, but every patient and situation is different. Estimates can bring both optimism and a sense of sadness to the caregiver and patient. You are better off to take advantage of each day you have and live it to the fullest with your loved one or friend. Two months could mean several months or may mean only one day.

Deep down I knew this day might come, but I was not ready for it. I do not remember much that was said after that. My mind was running in so many directions. How could I tell her? The kids would need to be told. Diana's parents would need to know.

The things that lay ahead seemed too difficult to contemplate. But I had no choice. The family looked to me for strength and leadership. I knew I must some- how determine who should know, in what order, and when. I had promised Diana that I would not keep bad news from her. *How and when should I tell her?*

Diana's parents had already planned to spend a few days with us and would arrive the next day on Friday. We had planned to have the entire family over for supper on Saturday evening. I thought it over and decided that Saturday evening would be the best time to break the news to the family. Diana was sleeping much of the time now. I would wait until she went to bed and then deliver the difficult news to the family.

As a caregiver, you may be confronted with the responsibility of bearing bad news to family or close friends. Determining the best time and place can be difficult. I would encourage you to do it as simply and quickly as possible. Most people want others to be honest and upfront with them. It will be hard, but trying to keep it a secret may be even harder. Especially with those who know you best. They may be able to sense that something is wrong, and keeping it from them may make it worse.

The next couple of days seemed so long. I rehearsed how I would tell the family and changed the wording over and over in my mind. Saturday evening finally arrived. I prayed and asked God to guide my thoughts and give me words that would convey the necessary bad news and still have an underlying strength that would give a sense of God's peace and presence.

Diana retired early. The men were upstairs and the ladies downstairs. We could not all congregate upstairs and leave Diana alone downstairs, and we could not all gather downstairs, fearing that Diana might be awakened and overhear the conversation. Dorene told the ladies while I told the men. There were looks of shock and tears of sadness. We consoled each other as best we could. Dorene agreed to tell the rest of Diana's side of the family, and I would tell my side.

We shared with the family our plans for

informing Diana of what the future seemed to hold for her. We also asked them not to say anything to her about what they had just learned until we had the chance to share with her.

It was done. With one huge hurdle crossed, my thoughts began to drift again toward the week to come. *How will I tell Diana?* She had asked me only a few weeks earlier if I thought she was going to make it. How could I find the words? How could I keep my composure? How would she take it? How and when would be the best time?

I had asked the surgeon if there was any benefit for a new round of chemotherapy scheduled to begin Tuesday. He said the chemotherapy would be of no benefit in Diana's condition and would only make things harder for her during her last days.

I called Dr. Yardley's office, and we discussed Diana's future treatment. We agreed we would not move forward with any more treatment and that Diana should be told of her condition as soon as possible. We agreed it would be easier if it were done during the Tuesday visit. Dr. Yardley agreed to break the news to Diana.

Dorene accompanied us to Tennessee Oncology.

We were directed to the same examining room in which we had begun this difficult journey almost three years earlier. Dr. Yardley walked into the room. It was obvious that her demeanor was different than it had been on our previous visits.

During her examination, Diana brought up the subject of a new round of chemotherapy. The doctor was having difficulty finding the words to tell Diana that future treatment was futile. Dr. Yardley told Diana her condition had worsened and the future did not look good.

Diana sensed what was happening and tried to make it easier for Dr. Yardley. She immediately intervened and asked how long she might live with the chemo- therapy and how long without it. Dr. Yardley responded, "Possibly six months with the chemotherapy and only a couple of months at the most without it."

The doctor had tears in her eyes. The nurse was wiping her eyes. Dorene and I both were fighting to keep our composure. Diana told the doctor that further treatment was not necessary, that she did not want to experience what further treatment would bring.

She was more concerned at that point with making the doctor and those around her feel better than fretting about what she had just learned. She thanked Dr. Yardley and the nurse for all they'd done to help her. She was gracious and kind. She told them that the Lord was in control and that she had no fear of what lay ahead.

I remember the sorrow I felt in my heart at that moment. I did not feel it for myself, but thought of the devastating news Diana had just received. She had just been told that she had two months or less to live. I could only imagine how that kind of news would make one stop and pause at the thought of dying.

I again realized that this moment was bigger than me. God was the only one who could help Diana. I can't find the words to describe how wonderfully God's huge presence filled that small examining room. Instead of a time of deep sadness and hopelessness, it became a time of calmness and a warm sense of God's peace. Dr. Yardley and her top nurse left the room having been impacted in a great way by Diana's strong positive reaction to the worst news they could have possibly brought and three years worth of a godly life lived before them. They will never be the same.

I ran into Dr. Yardley about two years later in an airport while on a business trip. She saw me before I saw her and approached me wanting to know how I was doing. I told her how God had blessed me and that I was doing well. She brought up Diana at that point and complimented her highly on what a fighter she had been and such a ne Christian lady. I could tell that Diana's testimony was still having an impact on her life.

Caregiver Principles

- There is a point in treatment when the reality of impending loss must be recognized and accepted.

- Honesty is the best policy. Respect your loved one's wishes to know.

- Difficult news must be carefully delivered.

- Determine how and when your loved one should be informed.

- Determine others who should know and in what order.

- Timing is important. When to inform the loved one and when to inform other family members should be carefully thought through.

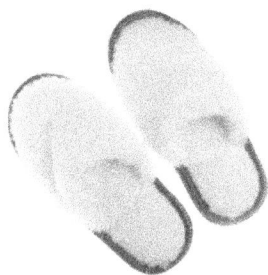

it hurts so badly

I dreaded the ride home. What could I say? How could I encourage her? I was truly amazed with what took place. Diana was more upbeat than she had been in a year. She knew the kids were coming over that evening, and she was excited about seeing them and the grandchildren. Her appetite had waned, but now she had a craving for pizza from Pizza Hut.

I had arranged for the entire family to eat supper together that evening. The kids knew their mom would find out about her impending death from the doctor, and we all wanted to be together to com- fort her and support each other. Diana laughed and played with the grandchildren. It was one of the most enjoyable evenings we'd experienced in a long time. She stayed up later than normal that evening and seemed to have a burst of energy that had not been present for several months.

Shortly after midnight, I was awakened by Diana's need to be helped to the restroom. I lifted her from bed and placed her in the wheelchair, taking care to position the oxygen line so we could make it easily to the restroom. I helped her get situated in the restroom and left the room with the door cracked to give her some privacy.

Preserving the privacy and dignity of a loved one or friend is important. As a caregiver, make every effort to be as sensitive as possible to this need. Being consider- ate and making the person you are giving care to feel comfortable will help them maintain that sense of personal privacy and dignity. Closing a door, using a sheet to provide modesty, turning a head while helping in and out of vehicles or furniture, along with other things will put the loved one or friend at ease and help them feel a certain sense of modesty and dignity.

Diana cried out and called my name. I quickly opened the door. "I cannot feel my legs," she said.

I was not overly alarmed because of previous occasions when a leg or arm would go to sleep. I helped her back into the wheelchair and back to the bed. I began to rub one leg and then the other to get the circulation moving again.

Dorene had decided to spend the night instead of

going home and was sleeping upstairs. I was so glad
that she had made that decision. She awoke to something happening downstairs. She quickly made her
way down the steps and into the room, and I told her
of the numbness. She began to help me rub Diana's
legs. In a few moments Diana's parents heard the
moans of pain and the frantic efforts to bring some
relief to her aching legs. They joined us as it became
obvious that the situation was not improving.

I called 911 and requested an ambulance. The
paramedics arrived within minutes and determined
quickly that she needed to be transported to the
hospital. Dorene agreed to ride with Diana in the
ambulance, and I would drive myself and Diana's
parents in our car.

We arrived a few minutes before the ambulance
and waited at the door of the emergency room as
Diana arrived. Diana's parents remained in the
waiting area, and Dorene and I stayed with Diana.

After the examination, the doctor wanted to talk
with me outside the room. I will always remember
the conversation that followed. The doctor began his
diagnosis. Diana had developed a blood clot in the
main artery that delivered blood flow to her lower
extremities. There was no blood owing to her legs. I

stood there stunned. I couldn't think. I remember asking him what it meant and what we could do.

"She is going to die," he said. "We could do surgery, but her physical condition is so bad she would not survive open heart surgery."

"Is there anything we can do?"

"We will make her as comfortable as possible, but nothing else can be done. She probably will not live through the night."

What should I do now? Diana's parents were in the waiting area. They needed to know. The children needed to know so they could spend those last few hours with their mom. Her siblings should know. My parents, my brother and his family, my church family all needed to know. My head was spinning. I knew deep down this day might come. I never dreamed it would arrive so quickly.

Dorene and I walked to the waiting area and sat down with Diana's parents. I tried to speak as tenderly and compassionately as I could. I relayed the diagnosis and told them the doctor said Diana was not going to make it. The sadness in their eyes was beyond description.

Dorene sat with her parents and tried to give them comfort. I could not sit with them very long because the children needed to know. I did not want to give the children such sad news on the phone. I stepped outside the emergency room waiting area to the parking lot and called both children. I asked them to come to Baptist Hospital as soon as they could because things did not look good for their mother.

Diana had not been told how serious things were. I felt as if the weight of the whole world was on my shoulders. How could I tell her she was about to die? I was about to lose the person who had been the love of my life for the past thirty-three years. I just could not be the one to do it.

I asked the doctor if he would tell Diana of her condition. He agreed but honored my request to wait until the children arrived. We gathered beside her bed as the doctor walked in. He got Diana's attention and began to tell her of the blood clot and what was happening to her body. He told her that nothing could be done and that she would not make it. My son broke down in the room. There were tears all around and a feeling of helplessness. We could do nothing, yet we had to do something.

Eventually it was determined that it would be

better to move Diana from the emergency room to a private room and make her as comfortable as possible there. A male nurse accompanied us as we made our way to the assigned room. We lost Diana in the hall- way, but the nurse was able to revive her. We eventually made it to a room around daybreak.

Diana took a turn for the better that would last most of the day. It didn't take long for word of her impending death to run the circuit throughout the city. She was loved by all who knew her. There was a continual flow of friends through Baptist Hospital. The day became more difficult as the minutes passed. It would be twenty-two hours from the first alarm until the final good-bye.

It's hard to describe what was going through my mind. Physically, I was tired. It had been over a year since I'd slept an entire night. I could sense the end was near for a relationship that had begun over thirty- four years ago. My thoughts were not of the past or the future but making sure she did not suffer now. Her death would come softly and peacefully.

The technicians placed a handheld pain-relief pump at Diana's side. Pain-relief medicine could be placed directly into her bloodstream every fifteen minutes. The doctors were amazed at how she was able to survive and remain conscious when her lower extremities were basically dead.

I sat by her bedside then moved across the room on the windowsill, leaving the room only briey a few times and then was back by her side. I had mixed feelings. She had suffered so much with this terrible disease.

Death was near. Selfishly, I could not imagine life without her, but I did not want her suffering to continue. My emotions moved into a feeling of numbness. I was involved in something I had absolutely no control over. God creates life, and all life belongs to him. The circle of life ends where it begins: in the hands of God. The circle of Diana's life was about to be completed.

The day continued to move forward—midmorning, noon, and three p.m. About six p.m. Diana slowly drifted off into unconsciousness. She lay there three to four more hours. Her room, the hallway, and waiting area down the hall were filled with family, friends, coworkers, and church members. Many had remained with us throughout the day and evening.

I'm not sure of the exact time, but around nine

thirty p.m. one of the most unusual things happened that I have ever witnessed. Diana awoke. She was completely conscious. She sat up quickly in the bed, gazing toward the ceiling. She had a glow about her that is impossible to adequately describe. She reached her arms toward heaven as if reaching to embrace someone. It was as though no one else was in the room. It was obvious she saw a heavenly being that was about to lift her into his arms and carry her across the deep, cold waters of death. She sat in that heavenly embrace for what seemed to be a long time but in reality was only a minute or so.

She slowly dropped her arms and lay back in the bed with her head turned and her eyes fixed on mine. I could not shift my eyes away from her gaze. I knew this was it. The time to say good-bye was now. As my heart was breaking, I watched the glow disappear from her face and the light of life in her eyes flicker dimly and finally go completely dark. The look of life and love was now a lifeless stare of death. I didn't know what to do or say. She was gone. I had other members of my family nearby, but I felt so alone.

Our family doctor Paul Gentuso, also a close friend, checked her vital signs then of officially let us know she was gone. He took his fingers, gently brushed them over her face, and closed her eyes.

There had been an abiding peace present in the room throughout the day, which now took on a much more prominent role. God reminds us in his Word that "the death of each of his saints is precious to him" (Psalm 116:15 nkjv). The presence of heaven was obvious and real in that room at that hour.

Then a strange thing happened. A spontaneous rendition of "Amazing Grace" swept across the room and down the hall. As we said good-bye, heaven said hello. We watched Diana lay down her suffering, cancer-ravaged body. Heaven welcomed her into the joy the Lord has prepared for those who love him. Suddenly, it was not a time of sadness but one of rejoicing. We knew it was not the end but only the beginning. She could not return to us, but we all could go to her. We would see her again.

Caregiver Principles

What had I learned over the past twenty-four hours? I was again reminded that God is in control in matters of life and death. The highest goal of men should be to honor God and bring praise to him through their lives. Only God knows how best this can be done.

We have our own ways of measuring success. We measure in goods accumulated and/or positions achieved. God's ways are not our ways. He is not impressed with our material goods. Everything on this earth is his anyway. "The earth is his and the full- ness thereof" (Psalm 24:1 nkjv).

His Word also teaches us that "in him all things consist *or exist*" (Colossians 1:17 nkjv). He is ruler of the universe. Can we impress him with achieving small recognitions by other men?

We follow his direction and example. "He was obedient unto death, even death on the cross" (Philippians 2:8 nkjv). The greatest achievement in life is surrendering our lives to him for his glory and praise.

He used Diana's life to impact so many others. She was a witness to many in the cancer-treatment facilities, hospital wards, and medical-testing facilities. She was obedient unto death, a death that if given the choice, most of us would not want to experience. She suffered willingly. She never wavered in her love for Christ and abiding resolution that this was what he had for her. She was faithful through the final hour. Her example was a shining testimony to her family, friends, church, and coworkers.

There is a time to hold onto loved ones with all the tenacity you possess. You want the best doctors, the latest medical procedures, and are even willing to try promising experimental drugs when all else fails. You spare no expense. You do battle with insurance companies to allow the treatment that medical professionals prescribe. You hold on because of hope of a cure. You are striving for healing so life can simply return to the way it was before the onslaught of the terrible disease.

There is also a time to let go. You will have help recognizing when that time arrives. I listened carefully to Diana's words, tone, and body language through- out the three years of the illness. It became obvious when Diana reached the conclusion that she would not get better. Her body had been battered with the disease and the chemicals to treat it. Her body was tired and worn out with the struggle. There was nothing left with which to fight. I could see that she saw the end approaching. She had fought a good fight, she was about to finish her course, and she had kept her faith. She knew the Lord had better things ahead than what she was experiencing here.

I could see it was time for me to let go. It would

be unfair to encourage her to continue suffering simply because the children and I did not want to live without her. I remember telling her in those last few minutes that it was okay to go on. I remember my son telling her, "Mom, we'll be okay. Go ahead and let go." I believe he was the last one she heard before she passed on. Letting go is not easy, but holding on can be even harder.

Learn the value of family and friends. They will be there in the beginning and remain until the end.

You can make it through hard and difficult days. God is faithful. Even though life seems so dark and cold at times, God will never leave you or forsake you.

then came the rainbow

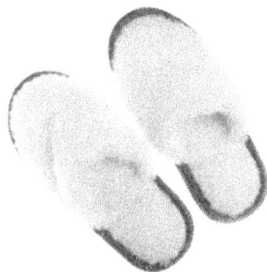

I remember receiving and reading a poem titled "A Road Less Traveled." It came at a dark and difficult time. I do not remember much about the words, but I identified with the concept. I am a few years removed from the loss of Diana and a few more than that since first receiving the news of her cancer.

It takes a period of time to regain perspective and refocus on life. That amount of time will be different for each individual. If you have recently lost someone for whom you were the caregiver, give life a little time. Time is a valuable ally. Time will help you reconstruct your life. I can see much more clearly now than during those early months after her passing.

The journey was so dark at times. I remember when I had prayed hard and fervently that God would heal and restore Diana. I almost became numb. I felt so beaten down and battered by life that prayer became more difficult. Many times in the last months of Diana's life I could only find words to beg God to help us.

Diana slept most of the time, and I felt so alone. The chemotherapy and cancer had affected her personality. I attended to her every need as best I could, but she was not herself. She couldn't help it, and I knew it.

She wanted to get a puppy. We'd had other dogs through the years, but I knew with her low resistance and the possible germs a dog might introduce that it would not be a good idea. I knew also I just could not take on anything more and that a puppy would require much time and attention. I remember her saying, "I want to get a puppy because I want something to need me."

My heart ached. Oh, how I needed her. Oh, how I longed for a gentle word or a loving touch. She did not realize how it sounded. At that point she was so sick she no longer could see much of what was going on in my personal world.

You may be experiencing this as a caregiver. You long for that loving touch or a gentle word. It can be a lonely time in your life. There is only one place of refuge that I found that can bring what you need. God is my refuge and strength, as the Holy Scriptures tell us, and he can be that for you. The kind word can be found by allowing him to speak to you through his Word.

Find time to read his Word each day. The book of Psalms is a great book of encouragement. You can also find a gentle touch through God's personal presence in your life. His Holy Spirit dwells in our hearts and brings a sense of personal peace. Look to God. Reach out to him. He does understand. He can help and will.

It is hard to believe she is gone. Her struggle is over and her victory is assured. But how can one go on? Those were dark days, and I could not understand how the sun could continue to rise in the morning. I was not suicidal, but I wanted the Lord to take me too.

I was all alone. Sure, I had family, friends, and my church family, but no one was there when I came home at night. There was no longer a need to call home when I was going to be late. The emptiness was beyond description.

Carrying my own grief and shouldering the

problems my church members faced were almost over- whelming at times. I had no one at home to support me or look after me. I remember one day in particular. It was our anniversary. It had been nine months since Diana's death, and Christmas was a week away. I remember visiting her grave and weeping. It had been nine months, and the pain should have been less. How could I face Christmas alone?

God did a work in my heart that day as I laid two dozen roses on the grave. He reminded me that he still had work for me to do. He had a plan for my life, just as he'd had a plan for Diana's life.

I didn't hear an audible voice. The men in white coats may come and get you if you acknowledge that. But it was as though he was telling me, "Roy, you've had almost a year now. You've made it through all the firsts except for a couple more. You've made it through Mother's Day, Father's Day, your birthday, her birth- day, Thanksgiving, and now your anniversary. Souls are at risk, and I have things for you to do. You *must* go on. You do have a life, and this sad time will pass.

As a caregiver, I want to alert you up front that the first year can be difficult. You will be confronted with all those *firsts*. Valentine's Day, Mother's Day, Father's Day, Fourth of July, the annual vacation to the mountains or beach, Labor Day, Thanksgiving, and Christmas can be hard days with the emptiness of missing that loved one or close friend. With each passing *first*, you will achieve a milestone. Try to alter the routine of those days to make them less difficult. Once you make it past that first year, the second year should be easier.

"You have followed me faithfully your entire adult life. I have not left you. I have not forsaken you. I have been faithful to you. Look at what you have around you. Look at your blessings. I have blessed you physically. You are healthy and have many years to live. I've blessed you personally. You have two wonderful children, who have ne Christian mates. You had three precious grandchildren before Diana's death, and I have given you another one during your time of grief. I've blessed you materially. Look at where you live, what you wear, how well you eat, and what you drive. I've even gone the extra mile and given you a Harley Davidson motorcycle to ride (just kidding). Look at how I've blessed you spiritually. You have a great church, and you've had great opportunities of service during your entire ministry."

God was letting me know that it was wrong for me to continue to focus on the hurt and the grief. I could no longer continue to remain in this state of sadness. Diana would not have wanted it. My children did not want it. But most importantly, God did not want it.

I talked to the Lord a great deal that day. I made a decision that with his help, I would do my best to move forward with my life. I would find the future by looking for him in the present. I determined that I would work on moving forward with my life one day at a time. I had spent almost four years taking life as it came, one day at a time.

God also has a plan for your life. Just as he has a plan for your loved one or friend, he has a future with your name on it. Take ample time to grieve after the one you have cared for passes on, but at some point you must move on with your life. You can do yourself harm and harm those who care about you by not coming to grips with your loss. It is not easy to move on, but it is even harder to stay in the depths of grief.

Make up your mind that you are going to live life one day at a time. Take it as it comes. The past no longer exists, and the future never arrives. It will always be today. Look for the future by living in the present. God has a great life in store for you. Your experiences will make you a more compassionate understanding person. God will use you to help others. Make the conscious decision to move on. Write down the date where you will see it from time to time under the statement: I said yes to myself and want to move on.

God has things for you to do. Family and friends are counting on you. Others whom you haven't met yet are depending on you. Your life is not over, it is just moving into a bright new beginning.

> Trust in the Lord with all your heart and lean not unto your own understanding, in all your ways acknowledge him and he will direct thy paths.   Proverbs 3:5–6, kjv

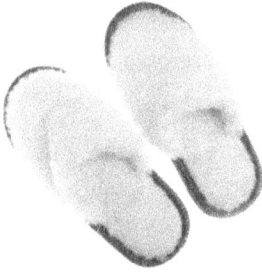

the final chapter

God's rainbow was the beginning of many new and exciting things he would send my way. He has restored my joy. He opened opportunities of service for me that had the potential of impacting thousands of lives. It was not so long ago I dreaded seeing the sun rise in the morning. Now I am excited about today and the future.

I have not found the pot of gold at the end of the rainbow yet, but I have found a beautiful rainbow at the end of a long, dark, and violent storm. I hear the birds singing again. I smell the pleasant fragrance of spring flowers and freshly cut grass. I notice the beautiful sunset.

Life is good. God is great. Will I ever completely get over the experience of losing a close loved one? I doubt it. The key is not trying to get completely over a tragic loss, but learning to live with and beyond it.

There is life after a great loss. One's personal

attitude greatly impacts what kind of life he or she will experience. You can choose to remain in the grip of grief, pain, and sorrow. It is not a great way to live. You will be sad and miserable and make others who love and care about you sad and miserable also.

You do have another choice. You can recognize that there are people who love and need you. They need you happy and contented. They need you upbeat and positive. They need you present and engaged with their lives.

You can make up your mind that with God's help you are going to move forward with your life. God has a plan for you just as he did for your dear loved one. It's his will for you to have joy and to find your place in life. Finding that plan begins with knowing him personally.
God has more in store for you.

Caregiver Principles

• Do not make rash emotional decisions during the first year.

• Do not make statements of what you will or will not do during the first few months. Those statements might ruin your opportunity for a happy future. Statements such as I'll never take this wedding ring off, I'll never date again, I'll never marry again, and I'll never live anywhere but in this house.